MedicalCenter.com

The Key Facts
On Coping With Cancer &
Cancer Resources

The Key Facts on Cancer: Volume VI

Everything You Need to Know About Coping With Cancer & Cancer Resources

-Usable Medical Information for the Patient-

By Patrick W. Nee

www.MedicalCenter.com

Published by:

MedicalCenter.com

96 Walter Street/ Suite 200

Boston, MA 02131, USA

Tel: 617-354-7722

www.MedicalCenter.com

manager@medicalcenter.com

The Key Facts on Cancer Series

<u>Table of Contents</u>

Chapter 1: Introduction

What is Cancer?

Cancer is a term used for diseases in which abnormal cells divide without control and are able to invade other tissues. Cancer cells can spread to other parts of the body through the blood and lymph systems.

Cancer is not just one disease but many diseases. There are more than 100 different types of cancer. Most cancers are named for the organ or type of cell in which they start - for example, cancer that begins in the colon is called colon cancer; cancer that begins in melanocytes of the skin is called melanoma.

Cancer types can be grouped into broader categories. The main categories of cancer include:

- *Carcinoma*- cancer that begins in the skin or in tissues that line or cover internal organs. There are a number of subtypes of carcinoma, including adenocarcinoma, basal cell carcinoma,squamous cell carcinoma, and transitional cell carcinoma.

- *Sarcoma* - cancer that begins in bone, cartilage, fat, muscle, blood vessels, or other connective or supportive tissue.

- *Leukemia* - cancer that starts in blood-forming tissue such as the bone marrow and causes large numbers of abnormal blood cells to be produced and enter the blood.
- *Lymphoma and myeloma* - cancers that begin in the cells of the immune system.
- *Central nervous system cancers* - cancers that begin in the tissues of the brain and spinal cord.

<u>Origins of Cancer</u>

All cancers begin in cells, the body's basic unit of life. To understand cancer, it's helpful to know what happens when normal cells become cancer cells.

The body is made up of many types of cells. These cells grow and divide in a controlled way to produce more cells as they are needed to keep the body healthy. When cells become old or damaged, they die and are replaced with new cells. However, sometimes this orderly process goes wrong. The genetic material (DNA) of a cell can become damaged or changed, producing mutations that affect normal cell growth and division. When this happens, cells do not die when they should and new cells form when the body does not need them. The extra cells may form a mass of tissue called a tumor.

Not all tumors are cancerous; tumors can be benign or malignant.

- **Benign tumors** aren't cancerous. They can often be removed, and, in most cases, they do not come back. Cells in benign tumors do not spread to other parts of the body.
- **Malignant tumors** are cancerous. Cells in these tumors can invade nearby tissues and spread to other parts of the body. The spread of cancer from one part of the body to another is called metastasis.

Some cancers do not form tumors. For example, leukemia is a cancer of the bone marrow and blood.

Cancer Statistics

A report from the nation's leading cancer organizations shows that rates of death in the United States from all cancers for men and women continued to fall between 2005 and 2009, the most recent reporting period available.

Estimated new cases and deaths from cancer in the United States in 2013:

- *New cases*: 1,660,290 (does not include nonmelanoma skin cancers)
- *Deaths*: 580,350

The risk of developing many types of cancer can be reduced by practicing healthy lifestyle habits, such as eating a healthy diet, getting regular exercise, and not smoking. Also, the sooner a cancer is found and treatment begins, the better the chances are that the treatment will be successful.

Chapter 2: Understanding Cancer Prognosis

- A prognosis is an estimate of the likely course and outcome of a disease.

- Many factors affect the prognosis of a person with cancer, including the type, location, and stage of the cancer.

- When estimating a patient's prognosis, doctors usually use statistics based on data from groups of people whose situations are most similar to that of the patient.

- Doctors cannot estimate with certainty what the outcome will be for an individual cancer patient.

What is a prognosis?

A prognosis is an estimate of the likely course and outcome of a disease. The prognosis of a patient diagnosed with cancer is often viewed as the chance that the disease will be treated successfully and that the patient will recover.

What factors affect a patient's prognosis?

Many factors can influence the prognosis of a person with cancer. Among the most important are the type and location of the cancer, the stage of the disease (the extent to which the cancer has spread in the body), and the cancer's grade (how abnormal the cancer cells look under a microscope—an indicator of how quickly the cancer is likely to grow and spread).

Other factors that affect prognosis include the biological and genetic properties of the cancer cells (these properties, which are sometimes called biomarkers, can be determined by specific lab and imaging tests), the patient's age and overall general health, and the extent to which the patient's cancer responds to treatment.

How do statistics contribute to predicting a patient's prognosis?

In estimating a cancer patient's prognosis, doctors consider the characteristics of the patient's disease, the available treatment options, and any health problems the patient may have that could affect the course of the disease or its ability to be treated successfully.

The doctor bases the prognosis, in large part, on information researchers have collected over many years about hundreds or even thousands of people with the same type of cancer.

When possible, doctors use statistics based on groups of people whose situations are most similar to that of the patient.

Several types of statistics may be used to estimate a cancer patient's prognosis. The most commonly used statistics are listed below.

- *Cancer-specific survival*: This statistic calculates the percentage of patients with a specific type and stage of cancer who have survived—that is, not died from—their cancer during a certain period of time (1 year, 2 years, 5 years, etc.) after diagnosis. Cancer-specific survival is also called disease-specific survival. In most cases, cancer-specific survival is based on causes of death in medical records, which may not be accurate. To avoid this inaccuracy, another method used to estimate cancer-specific survival that does not rely on information about the cause of death is relative survival.

- *Relative survival*: This statistic compares the survival of patients diagnosed with cancer (for example, breast cancer) with the survival of people in the general population who are the same age, race, and sex and who have not been diagnosed with that cancer. It is the percentage of cancer patients who have survived for a certain period of time after diagnosis relative to people without cancer.

- *Overall survival*: This statistic is the percentage of patients with a specific type and stage of cancer who are still alive—that is, have not died from any cause—during a certain period of time after diagnosis.

- *Disease-free survival*: This statistic is the percentage of patients who have no evidence of cancer during a certain period of time after treatment. Other similar terms are recurrence-free or progression-free survival.

Cancer survival statistics are frequently given in terms of 5-year survival relative to the general population (that is, as 5-year relative survival percentages or "rates"). For example, according to NCI's Surveillance, Epidemiology, and End Results program, the 5-year relative survival rate for all women diagnosed with breast cancer during the period from 2001 through 2007 was 89 percent and the 5-year relative survival rate for all patients diagnosed with lung cancer during the same period was 16 percent.

Because survival statistics are based on large groups of people, they cannot be used to predict exactly what will happen to an individual patient. No two patients are entirely alike, and their treatment and responses to treatment can vary greatly. Also, because it takes years to see the impact of new treatments and diagnostic tests, the statistics a doctor uses to make a prognosis may not reflect the effectiveness of current treatments.

Nevertheless, the doctor may speak of a favorable prognosis if the information from large groups of people suggests that the cancer is likely to respond well to treatment. A prognosis may be unfavorable if the cancer is likely to be difficult to control. It is important to keep in mind, however, that a prognosis is only an estimate. Again, doctors cannot be absolutely certain about the outcome for an individual patient.

Is it helpful to know the prognosis?

Cancer patients and their loved ones face many unknowns. Understanding their disease and what to expect can help patients and their loved ones make decisions about treatment, supportive and palliative care, rehabilitation, and personal matters, such as financial matters. Seeking information about prognosis is a personal decision.

Many people with cancer want to know their prognosis. They find it easier to cope when they know the likely course of their disease. Some patients may ask their doctor about survival statistics or search for this information on their own. Other people find statistical information confusing and frightening, and they think it is too impersonal to be of value to them. It is up to each patient to decide how much information he or she wants.

A doctor who is most familiar with a patient's situation is in the best position to discuss his or her prognosis and explain what the statistics may mean.

What is the prognosis if a patient decides not to have treatment?

Because everyone's situation is different, this question can be difficult to answer. Also, information used in making a prognosis often comes from studies that have compared new treatments with existing treatments rather than with "no treatment." Therefore, it is not always easy for doctors to accurately estimate the prognosis of a patient who decides not to have treatment. However, a doctor who is most familiar with a patient's situation is in the best position to discuss his or her prognosis.

There are many reasons why patients may decide not to have treatment. Some patients may be concerned that the benefits of cancer treatments will be outweighed by the side effects. Patients should discuss this concern with their doctor or other health care provider. Many medications are available to prevent or control the side effects caused by cancer treatments.

Some patients may decide at some point not to have treatment if they know that their type and stage of cancer has a poor prognosis, despite treatment. Patients who choose not to have active cancer treatment should talk with their doctor to ensure that they get palliative treatment to help with the symptoms caused by their disease.

In these cases, patients may want to think about clinical trials. Clinical trials are research studies that involve people. They test new ways to prevent, detect, diagnose, or treat diseases. People who take part in cancer clinical trials have an opportunity to contribute to scientists' knowledge about cancer and to help in the development of improved cancer therapies. They also receive state-of-the-art care from cancer experts.

What is the difference between a cure and a remission?

A cure means that treatment has successfully eradicated all traces of a person's cancer, and the cancer will never recur (return). A cure does not mean, however, that the person will never have cancer again. It is possible that another cancer, even the same type of cancer, will develop in the person's body at some point in the future.

A remission means that the signs and symptoms of a person's cancer are reduced. Remissions can be partial or complete. In a complete remission, all signs and symptoms of cancer have disappeared.

If a patient remains in complete remission for 5 years or more, some doctors may say that the patient is cured. However, some cancer cells can remain undetected in a person's body for years or even decades after apparently successful treatment, and these cells may eventually cause a recurrence. Although most types of cancer usually recur within the first 5 years after diagnosis and treatment, later recurrences always remain a possibility. Therefore, doctors cannot say with any certainty that an individual cancer patient is cured. The most they can say is that there are no signs of cancer at this time.

Because of the possibility of recurrence, doctors continue to monitor patients for many years and do tests to look for signs of cancer's return. They will also look for signs of delayed adverse effects from the cancer treatments received.

Chapter 3: Home Care for Cancer Patients

- Home care agencies may provide cancer patients with access to medical equipment; visits from registered nurses, physical therapists, and social workers; help with running errands, meal preparation, and personal hygiene; and delivery of medication.
- Medicare may offer reimbursement for some home care services. Medicaid covers part-time nursing care and home care aide services, as well as medical supplies and equipment.
- Veterans who are disabled as a result of military service can receive home care services from the U.S. Department of Veterans Affairs.

Why do some cancer patients choose home care?

Cancer patients often feel more comfortable and secure being cared for at home. Many patients want to stay at home so they will not be separated from family, friends, and familiar surroundings. Home care can help patients achieve this desire. It often involves a team approach that includes doctors, nurses, social workers, physical therapists, family members, and others.

Home care can be both rewarding and demanding for patients and caregivers. It can change relationships and require families to address new issues and cope with all aspects of patient care. To help prepare for these changes, patients and caregivers are encouraged to ask questions and get as much information as possible from the home care team or organizations devoted to home care. A doctor, nurse, or social worker can provide information about a patient's specific needs, the availability of home care services, and a list of local home care agencies.

What services are provided by home care agencies?

Services provided by home care agencies may include access to medical equipment; visits from registered nurses, physical therapists, and social workers; help with running errands, meal preparation, and personal hygiene; and delivery of medication. The state or local health department is another important resource in finding home care services. The health department should have a registry of licensed home care agencies.

How can cancer patients get assistance paying for home care?

Financial assistance to help patients pay for home care is available from public and private sources. The U.S. Department of Veterans Affairs (VA) and some government-sponsored programs, such as Medicare, Medicaid, and the Older Americans Act, cover home care for those who meet their criteria.

Some people may qualify for Medicare, a government health insurance program for the elderly or disabled that is administered by the Centers for Medicare & Medicaid Services (CMS). Cancer patients who qualify for Medicare may also be eligible for coverage or reimbursement of home hospice services if they are accepted into a Medicare-certified hospice program. Information is available at www.medicare.gov, from the toll-free Medicare hotline at 1–800–633–4227 (1–800–MEDICARE), or by writing to 7500 Security Boulevard, Baltimore, MD 21244–1850. Callers with TTY equipment may contact Medicare at 1–877–486–2048. The Home Health Compare website has information about Medicare-certified home health agencies and patients' rights.

Medicaid, a jointly funded, federal-state health insurance program for people who need financial assistance for medical expenses, is also coordinated by CMS. Coverage varies by state but may include part-time nursing care, home care aide services, and medical supplies and equipment. Information about coverage is available from local state welfare offices, state health departments, state social services agencies, or the state Medicaid office. Check the local telephone directory for the number to call

The Older Americans Act provides federal funds for state and local social service programs that help frail and disabled people age 60 and older remain independent. This funding covers home care aide, personal care, meal delivery, and escort and shopping services. Older persons, their caregivers, or anyone concerned about the welfare of an older person can contact their local Area Agency on Aging (AAA) for information and referrals to services and benefits in the community. AAAs are usually listed in the white pages of the phone book under the city or county government headings. The Eldercare Locator, which is operated by the U.S. Administration on Aging, provides information about AAAs and other assistance for older people. The Eldercare Locator can be reached at 1–800–677–1116.

Veterans who are disabled as a result of military service can receive home care services from the VA. Only home care services provided by VA hospitals may be used. More information about these benefits is available at 1–877–222–8387 (1–877–222–VETS).

Private health insurance policies may cover some home care or hospice services, but benefits vary from plan to plan. Policies generally pay for services given by skilled professionals, but the patient may be responsible for a deductible or co-payment. Many health maintenance organizations require that home care or hospice services be given by authorized agencies. Contact the insurance company to see which services are covered.

Many national organizations, such as the American Cancer Society (ACS), offer services to cancer patients and their families. Services vary among ACS chapters; however, many of the chapters can provide home care equipment or suggest other organizations that do. The ACS can be reached at 1–800–227–2345 (1–800–ACS–2345. For callers with TTY equipment, the number is 1–866–228–4327. The ACS also has fact sheets and materials about home care. Other voluntary agencies, such as the Red Cross and those affiliated with churches or social service organizations, may provide free or low-cost transportation. These agencies may also be able to lend home care equipment.

Chapter 4: Palliative Care in Cancer

- Palliative care is comfort care given to a patient who has a serious or life-threatening disease, such as cancer, from the time of diagnosis and throughout the course of illness. It is usually provided by a specialist who works with a team of other health care professionals, such as doctors, nurses, registered dieticians, pharmacists, and social workers.

- Palliative care is different from hospice care. Although they share the same principles of comfort and support, palliative care begins at diagnosis and continues during cancer treatment and beyond.

- Hospitals, cancer centers, and long-term care facilities provide palliative care. Patients may also receive it at home. Physicians and local hospitals can provide the names of palliative care or symptom management specialists.

- Palliative care addresses the emotional, physical, practical, and spiritual issues of cancer. Family members may also receive palliative care.

- Research shows that palliative care improves the quality of life of patients and family members, as well as the physical and emotional symptoms of cancer and its treatment.

What is palliative care?

Palliative care is care given to improve the quality of life of patients who have a serious or life-threatening disease, such as cancer. The goal of palliative care is to prevent or treat, as early as possible, the symptoms and side effects of the disease and its treatment, in addition to the related psychological, social, and spiritual problems. The goal is not to cure. Palliative care is also called *comfort care*, *supportive care*, and *symptom management*.

When is palliative care used in cancer care?

Palliative care is given throughout a patient's experience with cancer. It should begin at diagnosis and continue through treatment, follow-up care, and the end of life.

Who gives palliative care?

Although any medical professional may provide palliative care by addressing the side effects and emotional issues of cancer, some have a particular focus on this type of care. A palliative care specialist is a health professional who specializes in treating the symptoms, side effects, and emotional problems experienced by patients. The goal is to maintain the best possible quality of life.

Often, palliative care specialists work as part of a multidisciplinary team to coordinate care. This palliative care team may consist of doctors, nurses, registered dieticians, pharmacists, and social workers. Many teams include psychologists or a hospital chaplain as well. Palliative care specialists may also make recommendations to primary care physicians about the management of pain and other symptoms. People do not give up their primary care physician to receive palliative care.

If a person accepts palliative care, does it mean he or she won't get cancer treatment?

No. Palliative care is given in addition to cancer treatment. However, when a patient reaches a point at which treatment to destroy the cancer is no longer warranted, palliative care becomes the total focus of care. It will continue to be given to alleviate the symptoms and emotional issues of cancer. Palliative care providers can help ease the transition to end-of-life care.

What is the difference between palliative care and hospice?

Although hospice care has the same principles of comfort and support, palliative care is offered earlier in the disease process. As noted above, a person's cancer treatment continues to be administered and assessed while he or she is receiving palliative care. Hospice care is a form of palliative care that is given to a person when cancer therapies are no longer controlling the disease. It focuses on caring, not curing. When a person has a terminal diagnosis (usually defined as having a life expectancy of 6 months or less) and is approaching the end of life, he or she might be eligible to receive hospice care.

Where do cancer patients receive palliative care?

Cancer centers and hospitals often have palliative care specialists on staff. They may also have a palliative care team that monitors and attends to patient and family needs. Cancer centers may also have programs or clinics that address specific palliative care issues, such as lymphedema, pain management, sexual functioning, or psychosocial issues. A patient may also receive palliative care at home, either under a physician's care or through hospice, or at a facility that offers long-term care.

How does a person find a place that offers palliative care?

Patients should ask their doctor for the names of palliative care and symptom management specialists in the community. A local hospice may be able to offer referrals as well. Area hospitals or medical centers can also provide information. In addition, some national organizations have specific databases for referrals.

What issues are addressed in palliative care?

Palliative care can address a broad range of issues, integrating an individual's specific needs into care. The physical and emotional effects of cancer and its treatment may be very different from person to person. For example, differences in age, cultural background, or support systems may result in very different palliative care needs.

Comprehensive palliative care will take the following issues into account for each patient:

- *Physical.* Common physical symptoms include pain, fatigue, loss of appetite, nausea, vomiting, shortness of breath, and insomnia. Many of these can be relieved with medicines or by using other methods, such as nutrition therapy, physical therapy, or deep breathing techniques. Also, chemotherapy, radiation therapy, or surgery may be used to shrink tumors that are causing pain and other problems.

- *Emotional and coping.* Palliative care specialists can provide resources to help patients and families deal with the emotions that come with a cancer diagnosis and cancer treatment. Depression, anxiety, and fear are only a few of the concerns that can be addressed through palliative care. Experts may provide counseling, recommend support groups, hold family meetings, or make referrals to mental health professionals.

- *Practical.* Cancer patients may have financial and legal worries, insurance questions, employment concerns, and concerns about completing advance directives. For many patients and families, the technical language and specific details of laws and forms are hard to understand. To ease the burden, the palliative care team may assist in coordinating the appropriate services. For example, the team may direct patients and families to resources that can help with financial counseling, understanding medical forms or legal advice, or identifying local and national resources, such as transportation or housing agencies.

- *Spiritual.* With a cancer diagnosis, patients and families often look more deeply for meaning in their lives. Some find the disease brings them more faith, whereas others question their faith as they struggle to understand why cancer happened to them. An expert in palliative care can help people explore their beliefs and values so that they can find a sense of peace or reach a point of acceptance that is appropriate for their situation.

Can a family member receive palliative care?

Yes. Family members are an important part of cancer care, and, like the patient, they have a number of changing needs. It's common for family members to become overwhelmed by the extra responsibilities placed upon them. Many find it difficult to care for a relative who is ill while trying to handle other obligations, such as work and caring for other family members. Other issues can add to the stress, including uncertainty about how to help their loved one with medical situations, inadequate social support, and emotions such as worry and fear. These challenges can compromise their own health. Palliative care can help families and friends cope with these issues and give them the support they need.

How is palliative care given at the end of life?

Making the transition from curative treatment to end-of-life care is a key part of palliative care. A palliative care team can help patients and their loved ones prepare for physical changes that may occur near the end of life and address appropriate symptom management for this stage of care. The team can also help patients cope with the different thoughts and emotional issues that arise, such as worries about leaving loved ones behind, reflections about their legacy and relationships, or reaching closure with their life. In addition, palliative care can support family members and loved ones emotionally and with issues such as when to withdraw cancer therapy, grief counseling, and transition to hospice.

How do people talk about palliative care or decide what they need?

Patients and their loved ones should ask their doctor about palliative care. In addition to discussing their needs for symptom relief and emotional support, patients and their families should consider the amount of communication they need. What people want to know about their diagnosis and care varies with each person. It's important for patients to tell their doctor about what they want to know, how much information they want, and when they want to receive it.

Who pays for palliative care?

Palliative care services are usually covered by health insurance. Medicare and Medicaid also pay for palliative care, depending on the situation. If patients do not have health insurance or are unsure about their coverage, they should check with a social worker or their hospital's financial counselor.

Is there any research that shows palliative care is beneficial?

Yes. Research shows that palliative care and its many components are beneficial to patient and family health and well-being. A number of studies in recent years have shown that patients who have their symptoms controlled and are able to communicate their emotional needs have a better experience with their medical care. Their quality of life and physical symptoms improve.

In addition, the Institute of Medicine 2007 report Cancer Care for the Whole Patient cites many studies that show patients are less able to adhere to their treatment and manage their illness and health when physical and emotional problems are present.

Furthermore, patients who have serious illnesses and receive palliative care consultations have lower hospital costs than those who don't. These consultations help determine treatment priorities and, therefore, help patients avoid unnecessary tests and procedures.

Chapter 5: Hospice Care

- Hospice care focuses on controlling pain and other symptoms of illness so patients can remain as comfortable as possible near the end of life.

- Hospice care most often takes place at home, but it can also be provided in special in-patient facilities, hospitals, and nursing homes.

- To be eligible for hospice care under most insurance plans, patients must have a life expectancy of 6 months or less and sign a statement choosing hospice care. Hospice expenses may be covered by Medicare, Medicaid, or other health insurance plans.

What is hospice, and how is it used in cancer care?

Hospice is a special type of care in which medical, psychological, and spiritual support are provided to patients and their loved ones when cancer therapies are no longer controlling the disease. Hospice care focuses on controlling pain and other symptoms of illness so patients can remain as comfortable as possible near the end of life. Hospice focuses on caring, not curing. The goal is to neither hasten nor postpone death. If the patient's condition improves or the cancer goes into remission, hospice care can be discontinued and active treatment may resume. Choosing hospice care doesn't mean giving up. It just means that the goal of treatment has changed.

The hospice team usually includes doctors, nurses, home health aides, social workers, clergy or other counselors, and trained volunteers. The team may also include speech, physical, and occupational therapists, if needed. A hospice team member is on-call 24 hours a day, 7 days a week to provide support. The hospice team will work with the patient on the patient's goals for end-of-life care, not a predetermined plan or scenario. Hospice care is very individualized.

Hospice services may include doctor or nursing care, medical supplies and equipment, home health aide services, short-term respite (relief) services for caregivers, drugs to help manage cancer-related symptoms, spiritual support and counseling, and social work services. Patients' families are also an important focus of hospice care, and services are designed to give them assistance and support.

Hospice care most often takes place at home. However, hospice care can also be delivered in special in-patient facilities, hospitals, and nursing homes.

Who is eligible for hospice care?

Under most insurance plans in the United States, including Medicare, acceptance into hospice care requires a statement by a doctor and the hospice medical director that the patient has a life expectancy of 6 months or less if the disease runs its normal course. The patient also signs a statement saying that he or she is choosing hospice care. (Hospice care can be continued if the patient lives longer than 6 months, as long as the hospice medical director or other hospice doctor recertifies the patient's condition.)

The hospice team or insurance provider can answer questions about whether specific care decisions, such as getting a second opinion or participating in a clinical trial while in hospice care, would affect eligibility for hospice services.

How can people get help paying for hospice services?

Medicare and most Medicaid and private insurance plans cover hospice services.

Medicare is a government health insurance program for the elderly and disabled that is administered by the Centers for Medicare & Medicaid Services (CMS). The Medicare hotline can answer general questions about Medicare benefits and refer people to their regional home health intermediary for information about Medicare-certified hospice programs. The hotline number is 1–800–MEDICARE (1–800–633–4227); callers with TTY equipment can call 1–877–486–2048.

Medicaid, a federal-state partnership program that is part of CMS and is administered by each state, is designed for people who need financial assistance for medical expenses. Information about coverage is available from local state welfare offices, state public health departments, state social services agencies, or the state Medicaid office.

Information about the types of costs covered by a particular private policy is available from a hospital business office or hospice social worker, or directly from the insurance company.

Local civic, charitable, or religious organizations may also be able to help patients and their families with hospice expenses.

What is the difference between hospice and palliative care?

Although hospice and palliative care share the same principles of providing comfort and support for patients, palliative care is available throughout a patient's experience with cancer, whereas hospice is offered only toward the end of life. A person's cancer treatment continues to be administered and assessed while he or she is receiving palliative care, but with hospice care the focus has shifted to just relieving symptoms and providing support.

Where can people learn more about hospice?

The following organizations can provide more information about hospice.

National Hospice and Palliative Care Organization

>1–800–658–8898 (helpline)
>
>1–877–658–8896 (multilingual line)
>
>caringinfo@nhpco.org
>
>www.caringinfo.org
>
>The National Hospice and Palliative Care Organization's Caring Connections website offers information and publications focused on improving end-of-life care for adults and children. The site includes a database of national hospice programs. Some Spanish-language publications are available.

Hospice Association of America

>202–546–4759
>
>www.nahc.org/HAA/home.html
>
>The Hospice Association of America distributes publications on such topics as the history of hospice, the benefits of hospice, hospice-related statistics, and locations of hospice organizations.

Hospice Education Institute

207–255–8800

1–800–331–1620

info@hospiceworld.org

www.hospiceworld.org

The Hospice Education Institute operates HOSPICELINK, a toll-free telephone service that provides referrals to hospice and palliative care programs in the United States. HOSPICELINK also provides information about the principles and practices of good hospice and palliative care.

Hospice Net

info@hospicenet.org

www.hospicenet.org

Hospice Net provides information and support to patients facing life-threatening illnesses and to their families and friends.

American Cancer Society

1–800–ACS–2345 (1–800–227–2345)

www.cancer.org

The American Cancer Society (ACS) provides free fact sheets and publications about hospice. The address of a local ACS chapter can be obtained by calling the organization's toll-free telephone number.

Chapter 6: End-of-Life Care for People Who Have Cancer

- End-of-life care provides physical, mental, and emotional comfort, as well as social support, to people who are living with and dying of advanced illness.
- People who have already discussed their wishes for end-of-life care with their loved ones feel less stress at the end of their life, and so do their families.
- Advance directives are legal documents that record a person's wishes for end-of-life care.
- Research has shown that hospice care may improve the quality of life of a cancer patient who is dying and of the patient's family.

What does end-of-life care mean for people who have cancer?

When a cancer patient's health care team determines that the cancer can no longer be controlled, medical testing and cancer treatment often stop. But the person's care continues, with an emphasis on improving their quality of life and that of their loved ones, and making them comfortable for the following weeks or months.

Medicines and treatments people receive at the end of life can control pain and other symptoms, such as constipation, nausea, and shortness of breath. Some people remain at home while receiving these treatments, whereas others enter a hospital or other facility. Either way, services are available to help patients and their families with the medical, psychological, social, and spiritual issues around dying. Hospice programs are the most comprehensive and coordinated providers of these services.

The period at the end of life is different for each person. The signs and symptoms people have vary as their illness continues, and each person has unique needs for information and support. Questions and concerns that family members have about the end of life should be discussed with each other, as well as with the health care team, as they arise. Communication about end-of-life care and decision making during the final months of a person's life are very important. Research has shown that if a person who has advanced cancer discusses his or her options for care with a doctor early on, that person's level of stress decreases and their ability to cope with illness increases. Studies also show that patients prefer an open and honest conversation with their doctor about choices for end-of-life care early in the course of their disease, and are more satisfied when they have this talk.

Experts strongly encourage patients to complete advance directives, which are documents stating a person's wishes for care. They also designate who the patient chooses as the decision-maker for their care when they are unable to decide. It's important for people with cancer to have these decisions made before they become too sick to make them. However, if a person does become too sick before they have completed an advance directive, it's helpful for family caregivers to know what type of care their loved one would want to receive.

How do doctors know how long a person will continue to live?

Patients and their family members often want to know how long a person who has cancer will continue to live. It's normal to want to be prepared for the future. But predicting how long someone will continue to live is a hard question to answer. A number of factors, including the type of cancer, its location, and whether the patient has other illnesses, can affect what will happen.

Although doctors may be able to estimate the amount of time someone will continue to live based on what they know about that person, they might be hesitant to do so. They may be concerned about over- or under-estimating the person's remaining life span. They also might be fearful of giving false hope or destroying a person's will to live.

When should someone call for professional help if they're caring for a person who has cancer at home?

People caring for patients at home should ask them if they're comfortable, if they feel any pain, and if they're having any other physical problems.

There may be times when the caregiver needs assistance from the patient's health care team. A caregiver can contact the patient's doctor or nurse for help in any of the following situations:

- The patient is in pain that is not relieved by the prescribed dose of pain medication.
- The patient is experiencing onset of new symptoms, such as nausea, vomiting, increasing confusion, anxiety or restlessness.
- The patient is experiencing symptoms that were previously well controlled.
- The patient shows discomfort, such as by grimacing or moaning.

- The patient is having trouble breathing and seems upset.
- The patient is unable to urinate or empty the bowels.
- The patient has fallen.
- The patient is very depressed or talking about committing suicide.
- The caregiver has difficulty giving medicines to the patient.
- The caregiver is overwhelmed by caring for the patient, is too sad, or is afraid to be with the patient.
- The caregiver doesn't know how to handle a certain situation.

Keep in mind that palliative care experts can be called upon by the patient's physician at any point in the person's illness to help with these issues. They are increasingly available not only in the hospital, but also in the outpatient setting.

When is the right time to use hospice care?

Many people believe that hospice care is only appropriate in the last days or weeks of life. Yet Medicare states that it can be used as much as 6 months before death is anticipated. And those who have lost loved ones say that they wish they had called in hospice care sooner.

Research has shown that patients and families who use hospice services report a higher quality of life than those who don't. Hospice care offers many helpful services, including medical care, counseling, and respite care. People usually qualify for hospice when their doctor signs a statement saying that patients with their type and stage of disease, on average, aren't likely to survive beyond 6 months.

What are some ways to provide emotional support to a person who is living with and dying of cancer?

Everyone has different needs, but some worries are common to most dying patients. Two of these concerns are fear of abandonment and fear of being a burden. People who are dying also have concerns about loss of dignity and loss of control. Some ways caregivers can provide comfort to a person with these worries are listed below:

- Keep the person company. Talk, watch movies, read, or just be with him or her.
- Allow the person to express fears and concerns about dying, such as leaving family and friends behind. Be prepared to listen.
- Be willing to reminisce about the person's life.

- Avoid withholding difficult information. Most patients prefer to be included in discussions about issues that concern them.
- Reassure the patient that you will honor advance directives, such as living wills.
- Ask if there is anything you can do.
- Respect the person's need for privacy.
- Support the person's spirituality. Let them talk about what has meaning for them, pray with them if they'd like, and arrange visits by spiritual leaders and church members, if appropriate. Keep objects that are meaningful to the person close at hand.

What other issues should caregivers be aware of?

It's just as important for caregivers to take care of their own health at this time. Family caregivers are affected by their loved one's health more than they realize. Taking care of a sick person often causes physical and emotional fatigue, stress, depression, and anxiety. Because of this, it's important for caregivers to take care of their own body, mind, and spirit. Helping themselves will give them more energy, help them cope with stress, and cause them to be better caregivers as a result.

It's also helpful if caregivers ask for support from friends and family members. Such help is important to help lessen the many tasks involved in taking care of a loved one who is sick or dying.

What are some topics patients and family members can talk about?

For many people, it's hard to know what to say to someone at the end of life. It's normal to want to be upbeat and positive, rather than talk about death. And yet, it's important to be realistic about how sick the person may be. Caregivers can encourage their loved one without giving false hope.

Although it can be a time for grieving and accepting loss, the end of life can also be a time for looking for meaning and rethinking what's important.

During this period, many people tend to look back and reflect on life, legacies created, and loved ones who will be left behind. Some questions to explore with a patient at the end of life are the following:

- What are the happiest and saddest times we have shared together?
- What are the defining or most important moments of our life together?
- What are we most proud of?

- What have we taught each other?

Patients with serious, life-threatening illness have stated that being positive or adding humor remains an important outlet for them. Even at this challenging moment, laughter may still be the best medicine.

How should caregivers talk to their children about advanced cancer?

Children deserve to be told the truth about a family member's prognosis so they can be prepared if their loved one dies. It's important to answer all of their questions gently and honestly so they don't imagine things that are worse than reality. They need to be reassured that they will be taken care of no matter what happens.

Caregivers need to be prepared to answer tough questions. To do this, they should know what their own feelings and thoughts are about the situation. They need to be able to show children how to hope for the best while preparing for and accepting that their loved one may die.

How does cancer cause death?

Every patient is different, and the way cancer causes death varies. The process can depend on the type of cancer, where it is in the body, and how fast it's growing.

For some people, the cancer can't be controlled anymore and spreads to healthy tissues and organs. Cancer cells take up the needed space and nutrients that the healthy organs would use. As a result, the healthy organs can no longer function. For other people, complications from treatment can cause death.

During the final stages of cancer, problems may occur in several parts of the body.

- *Digestive system*: If cancer is in the digestive system (e.g., stomach, pancreas, or colon), food or waste may not be able to pass through, causing bloating, nausea, or vomiting. If the cancer prevents food from being digested or absorbed, patients can also become malnourished.

- *Lungs*: If too little healthy lung tissue is left, or if cancer blocks off part of the lung, the person may have trouble breathing and getting enough oxygen. Or, if the lung collapses, it may become infected, which may be too hard for someone with advanced cancer to fight.

- *Bones*: If cancer is in the bones, too much calcium may go into the bloodstream, which can cause unconsciousness and death. Bones with tumors may also break and not heal.

- *Liver*: The liver removes toxins from the blood, helps digest food, and converts food into substances needed to live. If there isn't enough healthy liver tissue, the body's chemical balance is upset. The person may eventually go into a coma.

- *Bone marrow*: When cancer is in the bone marrow, the body can't make enough healthy blood cells. A lack of red blood cells will cause anemia, and the body won't have enough oxygen in the blood. A low white blood cell count will make it hard to fight infection. And a drop in platelets will prevent the blood from clotting, making it hard to control abnormal bleeding.

- *Brain*: A large tumor in the brain may cause memory problems, balance problems, bleeding in the brain, or loss of function in another body part, which may eventually lead to a coma.

In some cases, the exact cause can't be pinpointed and patients simply decline slowly, becoming weaker and weaker until they succumb to the cancer.

Again, every patient is different and all processes have different stages and rates in which they advance. And some conditions have treatments that can help slow the process or make the patient more comfortable. It's very important to keep having conversations with the patient's health care team.

What are the signs that death is approaching, and what can the caregiver do to make the person comfortable during this time?

Certain signs and symptoms can help a caregiver anticipate when death is near. They are described below, along with suggestions for managing them. However, each person's experience at the end of life is different. What may happen to one person may not happen for another. Also, the presence of one or more of these symptoms doesn't necessarily mean that the patient is close to death. A member of the health care team can give family members and caregivers more information about what to expect.

Withdrawal from friends and family:

> People often focus inward during the last weeks of life. This doesn't necessarily mean that patients are angry or depressed or that they don't love their caregivers. It could be caused by decreased oxygen to the brain, decreased blood flow, and/or mental preparation for dying.

They may lose interest in things they used to enjoy, such as favorite TV shows, friends, or pets.

Caregivers can let the patient know they are there for support. The person may be aware and able to hear, even if they are unable to respond. Experts advise that giving them permission to "let go" may be helpful. If they do feel like talking, they may want to reminisce about joys and sorrows, or tie up loose ends.

Sleep changes:

People may have drowsiness, increased sleep, intermittent sleep, or confusion when they first wake up.

Worries or concerns may keep patients up at night. Caregivers can ask them if they would like to sit in the room with them while they fall asleep.

Patients may sleep more and more as time passes. Caregivers should continue to talk to them, even if they're unconscious, for the patient may still hear them.

Hard-to-control pain:

It may become harder to control pain as the cancer gets worse. It's important to provide pain medication regularly. Caregivers should ask to see a palliative care doctor or a pain specialist for advice on the correct medicines and doses. It may be helpful to explore other pain control methods such as massage and relaxation techniques.

Increasing weakness:

Weakness and fatigue will increase over time. The patient may have good days and bad days, so they may need more help with daily personal care and getting around.

Caregivers can help patients save energy for the things that are most important to them.

Appetite changes:

As the body naturally shuts down, the person with cancer will often need and want less food. The loss of appetite is caused by the body's need to conserve energy and its decreasing ability to use food and fluids properly.

Patients should be allowed to choose whether and when to eat or drink. Caregivers can offer small amounts of the foods the patient enjoys. Since chewing takes energy, they may prefer milkshakes, ice cream, or pudding. If the patient doesn't have trouble with swallowing, offer sips of fluids and use a flexible straw if they can't sit up. If a person can no longer swallow, offer ice chips. Keep their lips moist with lip balm and their mouth clean with a soft, damp cloth.

Awareness:

Near the end of life, people often have episodes of confusion or waking dreams. They may get confused about time, place, and the identity of loved ones. Caregivers can gently remind patients where they are and who is with them. They should be calm and reassuring. But if the patient is agitated, they should not attempt to restrain them. Let the health care providers know if significant agitation occurs, as there are treatments available to help control or reverse it.

Sometimes patients report seeing or speaking with loved ones who have died. They may talk about going on a trip, seeing lights, butterflies, or other symbols of reality we can't see. As long as these things aren't disturbing to the patient, caregivers can ask them to say more. They can let them share their visions and dreams, not trying to talk them out of what they believe they see.

The dying process:

There may be a loss of bladder or bowel control due to the muscles relaxing in the pelvis. Caregivers should continue to provide clean, dry bedding and gentle personal care. They can place disposable pads on the bed under the patient and remove them when soiled. Also, due to a slowing of kidney function and/or decreased fluid intake, there may be a decrease in the amount of urine. It may be dark and smell strong.

Breathing patterns may become slower or faster, in cycles. The patient may not notice, but caregivers should let the doctor know if they are worried about the changes. There may be rattling or gurgling sounds that are caused by saliva and fluids collecting in the throat and upper airways. Although this can be very disturbing for caregivers, at this stage the patient is generally not experiencing any distress. Breathing may be easier if a person's body is turned to the side and pillows are placed behind the back and beneath the head. Caregivers can also ask the health care team about using a humidifier or external source of oxygen to make it easier for the patient to breathe, if the patient is short of breath.

Skin may become bluish in color and feel cool as blood flow slows down. This is not painful or uncomfortable for the patient. Caregivers should avoid warming the patient with electric blankets or heating pads, which can cause burns. However, they may keep the patient covered with a light blanket.

What are the signs that the person has died?

- The person is no longer breathing and doesn't have a pulse.
- Their eyes don't move or blink, and the pupils are dilated (enlarged). The eyelids may be slightly open.
- The jaw is relaxed and the mouth is slightly open.
- The body releases the bowel and bladder contents.
- The person doesn't respond to being touched or spoken to.
- The person's skin is very pale and cool to the touch.

What needs to be done after the person has died?

After the person has died, there is no need to hurry with arrangements. Family members and caregivers may wish to sit with the body, to talk, or to pray. When the family is ready, the following steps can be taken.

- Place the body on its back with one pillow under the head. If necessary, caregivers or family members may wish to put the person's dentures or other artificial parts in place.

- If the person is in a hospice program, follow the guidelines provided by the program. A caregiver or family member can request a hospice nurse to verify the death.

- Contact the appropriate authorities in accordance with local regulations. Contact the person's doctor and funeral home.

- When the patient's family members are ready, call other family members, friends, and clergy.

- Provide or obtain emotional support for family members and friends to cope with their loss.

Chapter 7: Psychological Stress and Cancer

- Psychological stress alone has not been found to cause cancer, but psychological stress that lasts a long time may affect a person's overall health and ability to cope with cancer.
- People who are better able to cope with stress have a better quality of life while they are being treated for cancer, but they do not necessarily live longer.

What is psychological stress?

Psychological stress describes what people feel when they are under mental, physical, or emotional pressure. Although it is normal to experience some psychological stress from time to time, people who experience high levels of psychological stress or who experience it repeatedly over a long period of time may develop health problems (mental and/or physical).

Stress can be caused both by daily responsibilities and routine events, as well as by more unusual events, such as a trauma or illness in oneself or a close family member. When people feel that they are unable to manage or control changes caused by cancer or normal life activities, they are in distress. Distress has become increasingly recognized as a factor that can reduce the quality of life of cancer patients. There is even some evidence that extreme distress is associated with poorer clinical outcomes. Clinical guidelines are available to help doctors and nurses assess levels of distress and help patients manage it.

How does the body respond during stress?

The body responds to physical, mental, or emotional pressure by releasing stress hormones (such as epinephrine and norepinephrine) that increase blood pressure, speed heart rate, and raise blood sugar levels. These changes help a person act with greater strength and speed to escape a perceived threat.

Research has shown that people who experience intense and long-term (i.e., chronic) stress can have digestive problems, fertility problems, urinary problems, and a weakened immune system. People who experience chronic stress are also more prone to viral infections such as the flu or common cold and to have headaches, sleep trouble, depression, and anxiety.

Can psychological stress cause cancer?

Although stress can cause a number of physical health problems, the evidence that it can cause cancer is weak. Some studies have indicated a link between various psychological factors and an increased risk of developing cancer, but others have not.

Apparent links between psychological stress and cancer could arise in several ways. For example, people under stress may develop certain behaviors, such as smoking, overeating, or drinking alcohol, which increase a person's risk for cancer. Or someone who has a relative with cancer may have a higher risk for cancer because of a shared inherited risk factor, not because of the stress induced by the family member's diagnosis.

How does psychological stress affect people who have cancer?

People who have cancer may find the physical, emotional, and social effects of the disease to be stressful. Those who attempt to manage their stress with risky behaviors such as smoking or drinking alcohol or who become more sedentary may have a poorer quality of life after cancer treatment. In contrast, people who are able to use effective coping strategies to deal with stress, such as relaxation and stress management techniques, have been shown to have lower levels of depression, anxiety, and symptoms related to the cancer and its treatment. However, there is no evidence that successful management of psychological stress improves cancer survival.

Evidence from experimental studies does suggest that psychological stress can affect a tumor's ability to grow and spread. For example, some studies have shown that when mice bearing human tumors were kept confined or isolated from other mice—conditions that increase stress—their tumors were more likely to grow and spread (metastasize). In one set of experiments, tumors transplanted into the mammary fat pads of mice had much higher rates of spread to the lungs and lymph nodes if the mice were chronically stressed than if the mice were not stressed. Studies in mice and in human cancer cells grown in the laboratory have found that the stress hormone norepinephrine, part of the body's fight-or-flight response system, may promote angiogenesis and metastasis.

In another study, women with triple-negative breast cancer who had been treated with neoadjuvant chemotherapy were asked about their use of beta blockers, which are medications that interfere with certain stress hormones, before and during chemotherapy. Women who reported using beta blockers had a better chance of surviving their cancer treatment without a relapse than women who did not report beta blocker use. There was no difference between the groups, however, in terms of overall survival.

Although there is still no strong evidence that stress directly affects cancer outcomes, some data do suggest that patients can develop a sense of helplessness or hopelessness when stress becomes overwhelming. This response is associated with higher rates of death, although the mechanism for this outcome is unclear. It may be that people who feel helpless or hopeless do not seek treatment when they become ill, give up prematurely on or fail to adhere to potentially helpful therapy, engage in risky behaviors such as drug use, or do not maintain a healthy lifestyle, resulting in premature death.

How can people who have cancer learn to cope with psychological stress?

Emotional and social support can help patients learn to cope with psychological stress. Such support can reduce levels of depression, anxiety, and disease- and treatment-related symptoms among patients. Approaches can include the following:

- Training in relaxation, meditation, or stress management
- Counseling or talk therapy

- Cancer education sessions
- Social support in a group setting
- Medications for depression or anxiety
- Exercise

Some expert organizations recommend that all cancer patients be screened for distress early in the course of treatment. A number also recommend re-screening at critical points along the course of care. Health care providers can use a variety of screening tools, such as a distress scale or questionnaire, to gauge whether cancer patients need help managing their emotions or with other practical concerns. Patients who show moderate to severe distress are typically referred to appropriate resources, such as a clinical health psychologist, social worker, chaplain, or psychiatrist.

Chapter 8: How To Find a Doctor or Treatment Facility If You Have Cancer

- If you have been diagnosed with cancer, finding a doctor and treatment facility for your cancer care is an important step to getting the best treatment possible.

- Although the health care system is complex, resources are available to guide you in finding a doctor, getting a second opinion, and choosing a treatment facility.

How are doctors trained and certified to treat cancer patients?

When choosing a doctor for your cancer care, you may find it helpful to know some of the terms used to describe a doctor's training and credentials. Most physicians who treat people with cancer are medical doctors (they have an M.D. degree) or osteopathic doctors (they have a D.O. degree). The basic training for both types of physicians includes 4 years of premedical education at a college or university, 4 years of medical school to earn an M.D. or D.O. degree, and postgraduate medical education through internships and residences. This training usually lasts 3 to 7 years. Physicians must pass an exam to become licensed (legally permitted) to practice medicine in their state. Each state or territory has its own procedures and general standards for licensing physicians.

Specialists are physicians who have completed their residency training in a specific area, such as internal medicine. Independent specialty boards certify physicians after they have fulfilled certain requirements. These requirements include meeting specific education and training criteria, being licensed to practice medicine, and passing an examination given by the specialty board. Doctors who have met all of the requirements are given the status of "Diplomate" and are board certified as specialists. Doctors who are board eligible have obtained the required education and training but have not completed the specialty board examination.

After being trained and certified as a specialist, a physician may choose to become a subspecialist. A subspecialist has at least 1 additional year of full-time education in a particular area of a specialty. This training is designed to increase the physician's expertise in a specific field. Specialists can be board certified in their subspecialty as well.

The following are some specialties and subspecialties that pertain to cancer treatment:

- *Medical Oncology* is a subspecialty of internal medicine. Doctors who specialize in internal medicine treat a wide range of medical problems. Medical oncologists treat cancer and manage the patient's course of treatment. A medical oncologist may also consult with other physicians about the patient's care or refer the patient to other specialists.

- *Hematology* is a subspecialty of internal medicine. Hematologists focus on diseases of the blood and related tissues, including the bone marrow, spleen, and lymph nodes.

- *Radiation Oncology* is a subspecialty of radiology. Radiology is the use of x-rays and other forms of radiation to diagnose and treat disease. Radiation oncologists specialize in the use of radiation to treat cancer.

- *Surgery* is a specialty that pertains to the treatment of disease by surgical operation. General surgeons perform operations on almost any area of the body. Physicians can also choose to specialize in a certain type of surgery; for example, thoracic surgeons are specialists who perform operations specifically in the chest area, including the lungs and the esophagus.

The American Board of Medical Specialties® (ABMS) is a not-for-profit organization that assists medical specialty boards with the development and use of standards for evaluation and certification of physicians. Information about other specialties that treat cancer is available from the ABMS website www.abms.org.

Almost all board-certified specialists are members of their medical specialty society. Physicians can attain Fellowship status in a specialty society, such as the American College of Surgeons (ACS), if they demonstrate outstanding achievement in their profession. Criteria for Fellowship status may include the number of years of membership in the specialty society, years practicing in the specialty, and professional recognition by peers.

How can I find a doctor who specializes in cancer care?

One way to find a doctor who specializes in cancer care is to ask for a referral from your primary care physician. You may know a specialist yourself, or through the experience of a family member, coworker, or friend.

The following resources may also be able to provide you with names of doctors who specialize in treating specific diseases or conditions. However, these resources may not have information about the quality of care that the doctors provide.

- Your local hospital or its patient referral service may be able to provide you with a list of specialists who practice at that hospital.

- Your nearest NCI-designated cancer center can provide information about doctors who practice at that center.

- The ABMS has a list of doctors who have met certain education and training requirements and have passed specialty examinations. Is Your Doctor Board Certified lists doctors' names along with their specialty and their educational background. The directory is available in most libraries. www.certificationmatters.org

- The American Medical Association (AMA) DoctorFinder database provides basic information on licensed physicians in the United States. Users can search for physicians by name or by medical specialty. www.extapps.ama-assn.org/doctorfinder

- The American Society of Clinical Oncology (ASCO) provides an online list of doctors who are members of ASCO. The member database has the names and affiliations of nearly 30,000 oncologists worldwide. It can be searched by doctor's name, institution, location, oncology specialty, and/or type of board certification. www.cancer.net/all-about-cancer/newly-diagnosed/find-oncologist/find-oncologist-database
- The American College of Surgeons (ACS) membership database is an online list of surgeons who are members of the ACS. The list can be searched by doctor's name, geographic location, or medical specialty. The ACS can be contacted by telephone at 1–800–621–4111. www.web2.facs.org/acdir/default_public.cfm
- The American Osteopathic Association (AOA) Find a Doctor database provides an online list of practicing osteopathic physicians who are AOA members. The information can be searched by doctor's name, geographic location, or medical specialty. The AOA can be contacted by telephone at 1–800–621–1773.

www.osteopathic.org/osteopathic-health/find-a-do/Pages/default.aspx

- Local medical societies may maintain lists of doctors in each specialty.
- Public and medical libraries may have print directories of doctors' names listed geographically by specialty.
- Your local Yellow Pages or Yellow Book may have doctors listed by specialty under "Physicians."

If you are a member of a health insurance plan, your choice may be limited to doctors who participate in your plan. Your insurance company can provide you with a list of participating primary care doctors and specialists. It is important to ask whether the doctor you are considering is accepting new patients through your health plan. You also have the option of seeing a doctor outside your health plan and paying the costs yourself. If you have the option to change health insurance plans, you may first wish to consider which doctor or doctors you would like to use, and then choose a plan that includes your chosen physician(s).

If you are using a federal or state health insurance program such as Medicare or Medicaid, you may want to ask whether the doctor you are considering is accepting patients who use these programs.

You will have many factors to consider when choosing a doctor. To make an informed decision, you may wish to speak with several doctors before choosing one. When you meet with each doctor, you might want to consider the following:

- Does the doctor have the education and training to meet my needs?
- Does the doctor use the hospital that I have chosen?
- Does the doctor listen to me and treat me with respect?
- Does the doctor explain things clearly and encourage me to ask questions?
- What are the doctor's office hours?
- Who covers for the doctor when he or she is unavailable? Will that person have access to my medical records?
- How long does it take to get an appointment with the doctor?

If you are choosing a surgeon, you may wish to ask additional questions about the surgeon's background and experience with specific procedures. These questions may include:

- Is the surgeon board certified?
- Has the surgeon been evaluated by a national professional association of surgeons, such as the ACS?
- At which treatment facility or facilities does the surgeon practice?
- How often does the surgeon perform the type of surgery I need?
- How many of these procedures has the surgeon performed? What was the success rate?

It is important for you to feel comfortable with the specialist that you choose because you will be working closely with that person to make decisions about your cancer treatment. Trust your own observations and feelings when deciding on a doctor for your medical care.

How can I get another doctor's opinion about the diagnosis and treatment plan?

After your doctor gives you advice about the diagnosis and treatment plan, you may want to get another doctor's opinion before you begin treatment. This is known as getting a second opinion. You can do this by asking another specialist to review all of the materials related to your case. The doctor who gives the second opinion can confirm or suggest modifications to your doctor's proposed treatment plan, provide reassurance that you have explored all of your options, and answer any questions you may have.

Getting a second opinion is done frequently, and most physicians welcome another doctor's views. In fact, your doctor may be able to recommend a specialist for this consultation. However, some people find it uncomfortable to request a second opinion. When discussing this issue with your doctor, it may be helpful to express satisfaction with your doctor's decision and care and to mention that you want your decision about treatment to be as thoroughly informed as possible. You may also wish to bring a family member along for support when asking for a second opinion. It is best to involve your doctor in the process of getting a second opinion, because your doctor will need to make your medical records (such as your test results and x-rays) available to the specialist who is giving the second opinion.

Some health care plans require a second opinion, particularly if a doctor recommends surgery. Other health care plans will pay for a second opinion if the patient requests it. If your plan does not cover a second opinion, you can still obtain one if you are willing to cover the cost.

How can U.S. residents find treatment facilities?

Choosing a treatment facility is another important consideration for getting the best medical care possible. Although you may not be able to choose which hospital treats you in an emergency, you can choose a facility for scheduled and ongoing care. If you have already found a doctor for your cancer treatment, you may need to choose a facility based on where your doctor practices. Your doctor may be able to recommend a facility that provides quality care to meet your needs. You may wish to ask the following questions when considering a treatment facility:

- Has the facility had experience and success in treating my condition?
- Has the facility been rated by state, consumer, or other groups for its quality of care?
- How does the facility check on and work to improve its quality of care?
- Has the facility been approved by a nationally recognized accrediting body, such as the ACS Commission on Cancer and/or The Joint Commission?

- Does the facility explain patients' rights and responsibilities? Are copies of this information available to patients?
- Does the treatment facility offer support services, such as social workers and resources, to help me find financial assistance if I need it?
- Is the facility conveniently located?

If you are a member of a health insurance plan, your choice of treatment facilities may be limited to those that participate in your plan. Your insurance company can provide you with a list of approved facilities. Although the costs of cancer treatment can be very high, you do have the option of paying out-of-pocket if you want to use a treatment facility that is not covered by your insurance plan. If you are considering paying for treatment yourself, you may wish to discuss the possible costs with your doctor beforehand. You may also want to speak with the person who does the billing for the treatment facility. Nurses and social workers may also be able to provide you with more information about coverage, eligibility, and insurance issues.

The following resources may help you find a hospital or treatment facility for your care:

- The NCI-Designated Cancer Centers Find a Cancer Center page provides contact information for NCI-designated cancer centers located throughout the country. www.cancer.gov/researchandfunding/extramural/cancercenters/find-a-cancer-center

- The ACS's Commission on Cancer (CoC) accredits cancer programs at hospitals and other treatment facilities. More than 1,430 programs in the United States have been designated by the CoC as Approved Cancer Programs. The ACS website offers a searchable database of these programs. The CoC can also be contacted by telephone at 312–202–5085 or by e-mail at CoC@facs.org. www.datalinks.facs.org/cpm/cpmapprovedhospitals_search.htm

- The Joint Commission is an independent not-for-profit organization that evaluates and accredits health care organizations and programs in the United States. It also offers information for the general public about choosing a treatment facility. The Joint Commission can be contacted by telephone at 630–792–5000. www.jointcommission.org

The Joint Commission offers an online Quality Check® service that patients can use to determine whether a specific facility has been accredited by the Joint Commission and to view the organization's performance reports. www.qualitycheck.org/consumer/searchQCR.asp x

How can people who live outside the United States find treatment facilities in or near their countries?

If you live outside the United States, facilities that offer cancer treatment may be located in or near your country. Cancer information services are available in many countries to provide information and answer questions about cancer; they may also be able to help you find a cancer treatment facility close to where you live. A list of these cancer information services is available on the website of the International Cancer Information Service Group , an independent international organization of cancer information services. www.icisg.org/meet_memberslist.htm

A list may also be requested by writing to the NCI Public Inquiries Office at:

Cancer Information Service

Suite 300

6116 Executive Boulevard

Bethesda, MD 20892–8322

USA

The Union for International Cancer Control (UICC) is another resource for people living outside the United States who want to find a cancer treatment facility. The UICC consists of international cancer-related organizations devoted to the worldwide fight against cancer. UICC membership includes research facilities and treatment centers and, in some countries, ministries of health. Other members include volunteer cancer leagues, associations, and societies. These organizations serve as resources for the public and may have helpful information about cancer and treatment facilities. To find a resource in or near your country, contact the UICC at:

Union for International Cancer Control (UICC)

62 route de Frontenex

1207 Geneva

Switzerland

+ 41 22 809 1811

www.uicc.org

How can people who live outside the United States get a second opinion or have cancer treatment in the United States?

Some people living outside the United States may wish to obtain a second opinion or have their cancer treatment in this country. Many facilities in the United States offer these services to international cancer patients. These facilities may also provide support services, such as language interpretation, assistance with travel, and guidance in finding accommodations near the treatment facility for patients and their families.

If you live outside the United States and would like to obtain cancer treatment in this country, you should contact cancer treatment facilities directly to find out whether they have an international patient office. The NCI-Designated Cancer Centers Find a Cancer Center page offers contact information for NCI-designated cancer centers throughout the United States.

http://www.cancer.gov/researchandfunding/extramural/cancercenters/find-a-cancer-center

Citizens of other countries who are planning to travel to the United States for cancer treatment generally must first obtain a nonimmigrant visa for medical treatment from the U.S. Embassy or Consulate in their home country. Visa applicants must demonstrate that the purpose of their trip is to enter the United States for medical treatment; that they plan to remain for a specific, limited period; that they have funds to cover expenses in the United States; that they have a residence and social and economic ties outside the United States; and that they intend to return to their home country.

To determine the specific fees and documentation required for the nonimmigrant visa and to learn more about the application process, contact the U.S. Embassy or Consulate in your home country. A list of links to the websites of U.S. Embassies and Consulates worldwide can be found on the U.S. Department of State's website:

http://www.usembassy.gov

More information about nonimmigrant visa services is available on the U.S. Department of State's Temporary Visitors to the U.S. page:

www.travel.state.gov/visa/temp/temp_1305.html

Chapter 9: How To Find Resources in Your Own Community If You Have Cancer

- If you have cancer or are undergoing cancer treatment, there are places in your community to turn to for help. There are many local organizations throughout the country that offer a variety of practical and support services to people with cancer. However, people often don't know about these services or are unable to find them. National cancer organizations can assist you in finding these resources, and there are a number of things you can do for yourself.

- Whether you are looking for a support group, counseling, advice, financial assistance, transportation to and from treatment, or information about cancer, most neighborhood organizations, local health care providers, or area hospitals are a good place to start. Often, the hardest part of looking for help is knowing the right questions to ask.

What Kind of Help Can I Get?

Until now, you probably never thought about the many issues and difficulties that arise with a diagnosis of cancer. There are support services to help you deal with almost any type of problem that might occur. The first step in finding the help you need is knowing what types of services are available. The following pages describe some of these services and how to find them.

Information on Cancer

Most national cancer organizations provide a range of information services, including materials on different types of cancer, treatments, and treatment-related issues.

Counseling

While some people are reluctant to seek counseling, studies show that having someone to talk to reduces stress and helps people both mentally and physically. Counseling can also provide emotional support to cancer patients and help them better understand their illness. Different types of counseling include individual, group, family, self-help (sometimes called peer counseling), bereavement, patient-to-patient, and sexuality.

Medical Treatment Decisions

Often, people with cancer need to make complicated medical decisions. Many organizations provide hospital and physician referrals for second opinions and information on clinical trials (research studies with people), which may expand treatment options.

Prevention and Early Detection

While cancer prevention may never be 100 percent effective, many things (such as quitting smoking and eating healthy foods) can greatly reduce a person's risk for developing cancer. Prevention services usually focus on smoking cessation and nutrition. Early detection services, which are designed to detect cancer when a person has no symptoms of disease, can include referrals for screening mammograms, Pap tests, or prostate exams.

Home Health Care

Home health care assists patients who no longer need to stay in a hospital or nursing home, but still require professional medical help. Skilled nursing care, physical therapy, social work services, and nutrition counseling are all available at home.

Hospice Care

Hospice is care focused on the special needs of terminally ill cancer patients. Sometimes called palliative care, it centers around providing comfort, controlling physical symptoms, and giving emotional support to patients who can no longer benefit from curative treatment. Hospice programs provide services in various settings, including the patient's home, hospice centers, hospitals, or skilled nursing facilities. Your doctor or social worker can provide a referral for these services.

Rehabilitation

Rehabilitation services help people adjust to the effects of cancer and its treatment. Physical rehabilitation focuses on recovery from the physical effects of surgery or the side effects associated with chemotherapy. Occupational or vocational therapy helps people readjust to everyday routines, get back to work, or find employment.

Advocacy

Advocacy is a general term that refers to promoting or protecting the rights and interests of a certain group, such as cancer patients. Advocacy groups may offer services to assist with legal, ethical, medical, employment, legislative, or insurance issues, among others. For instance, if you feel your insurance company has not handled your claim fairly, you may want to advocate for a review of its decision.

Financial

Having cancer can be a tremendous financial burden to cancer patients and their families. There are programs sponsored by the Government and nonprofit organizations to help cancer patients with problems related to medical billing, insurance coverage, and reimbursement issues. There are also sources for financial assistance, and ways to get help collecting entitlements from Medicaid, Medicare, and the Social Security Administration.

Housing/Lodging

Some organizations provide lodging for the family of a patient undergoing treatment, especially if it is a child who is ill and the parents are required to accompany the child to treatment.

Children's Services

A number of organizations provide services for children with cancer, including summer camps, make-a-wish programs, and help for parents seeking child care.

How do I find these services?

Often, the services that people with cancer are looking for are right in their own neighborhood or city. The following is a list of places where you can begin your search for help.

- The hospital, clinic, or medical center where you see your doctor, received your diagnosis, or where you undergo treatment should be able to give you information. Your doctor or nurse may be able to tell you about your specific medical condition, pain management, rehabilitation services, home nursing, or hospice care.

- Most hospitals also have a social work, home care, or discharge planning department. This department may be able to help you find a support group, a nonprofit agency that helps people who have cancer, or the government agencies that oversee Social Security, Medicare, and Medicaid. While you are undergoing treatment, be sure to ask the hospital about transportation, practical assistance, or even temporary child care. Talk to a hospital financial counselor in the business office about developing a monthly payment plan if you need help with hospital expenses.

- The public library is an excellent source of information, as are patient libraries at many cancer centers. A librarian can help you find books and articles through a literature search.

- A local church, synagogue, YMCA or YWCA, or fraternal order may provide financial assistance, or may have volunteers who can help with transportation and home care. Catholic Charities or the American Red Cross may also operate local offices. Some of these organizations may provide home care.

- Local or county government agencies may offer low-cost transportation (sometimes called para-transit) to individuals unable to use public transportation. Most states also have an Area Agency on Aging that offers low-cost services to people over 60. Your hospital or community social worker can direct you to government agencies for entitlements, including Social Security, state disability, Medicaid, income maintenance, and food stamps. (Keep in mind that most applications to entitlement programs take some time to process.) The federal government also runs the Hill-Burton program (1–800–638–0742), which funds certain medical facilities and hospitals to provide cancer patients with free or low-cost care if they are in financial need.

What questions should I ask to get the most from a service?

No matter what type of help you are looking for, the only way to find resources to fit your needs is to ask the right questions. When you are calling an organization for information, it is important to think about what questions you are going to ask before you call. Many people find it helpful to write out their questions in advance, and to take notes during the call. Another good tip is to ask the name of the person with whom you are speaking in case you have follow-up questions. Below are some of the questions you may want to consider if you are calling or visiting a new agency and want to learn about how they can help:

- How do I apply [for this service]?
- Are there eligibility requirements? What are they?
- Is there an application process? How long will it take? What information will I need to complete the application process? Will I need anything else to get the service?
- Do you have any other suggestions or ideas about where I can find help?

The most important thing to remember is that you will rarely receive help unless you ask for it. In fact, asking can be the hardest part of getting help. Don't be afraid or ashamed to ask for assistance. Cancer is a very difficult disease, but there are people and services that can ease your burdens and help you focus on your treatment and recovery.

Chapter 10: Advanced Directives

- It is important for family members and health care providers to know what kind of medical care a patient wants at the end of life. Advance directives, which include living wills and medical powers of attorney, are legal documents that record the patient's wishes for end-of-life care.

- Advance directives should be filled out while people are healthy, because doing so gives them time to think about the end-of-life care they would choose if they were unable to communicate their own wishes. It also allows time to discuss these wishes with loved ones.

- The laws regarding advance directives vary from state to state, so it is important to complete and sign advance directives for the state where the patient lives or expects to receive medical treatment. The resources described in Question 10 can provide information and guidance.

What are advance directives?

Advance directives are legal documents that allow people to communicate their decisions about medical care to family, friends, and health care professionals in the event that they are unable to make those decisions themselves—for example, due to being unconscious or in a coma. The two main types of advance directives are a living will and a medical power of attorney.

What is a living will?

In a living will, people indicate what kind of medical care, especially life-sustaining care, they would or would not like to receive if they become unable to speak for themselves. The most common types of care that are addressed in a living will include:

- The use of life-sustaining equipment (such as dialysis machines, ventilators, and respirators)
- "Do not resuscitate" (DNR) orders; that is, instructions not to use cardiopulmonary resuscitation (CPR) if breathing or heartbeat stops
- Artificial hydration and nutrition (tube feeding)
- Withholding food and fluids
- Organ and tissue donation

What is a medical power of attorney?*

A medical power of attorney is the advance directive that allows people to name another person to make decisions about their medical care if they are temporarily or permanently unable to communicate or make these decisions for themselves. (This document can also be known as a "health care proxy," "appointment of health care agent," or "durable power of attorney for health care.") The scope of a medical power of attorney is not limited to choices at the end of life but also includes decisions in other medical situations. Generally, with a medical power of attorney, people appoint someone they know well and trust to carry out their wishes. This person may also be known as a health care agent, surrogate, attorney-in-fact, or health care proxy. The document goes into effect when a doctor declares that a person is unable to make his or her own medical decisions.

Why are advance directives important?

People have the right to make decisions about their own treatment. Filling out advance directives gives them a way to do so. Choices about end-of-life care can be difficult to make even when people are healthy, but if they are already seriously ill such decisions can seem overwhelming. Some cancer patients want to try every drug or treatment in the hope that something will be effective. Others will choose to stop anticancer therapy. Although patients may turn to family and friends for advice, ultimately it is the patient's decision.

It's important to keep in mind that when patients choose not to receive or to stop treatment to control the disease, medical care to promote their well-being (palliative care) continues. This type of care includes treatment to manage pain and other physical symptoms, as well as support for the psychosocial and spiritual needs of patients and their families.

When should people complete advance directives?

Many people associate advance directives with decisions made near the end of life. Yet, ideally, these documents should be completed while a person is healthy. People don't need to wait until they have been diagnosed with a serious illness to think through their wishes for care. In fact, making these choices when people are well can reduce the burden on them and their loved ones later on. Earlier communication ensures that patients with cancer or another serious disease will face the end of their lives with dignity and with treatment that reflects the values by which they have lived. As people prepare their advance directives, they should talk about their decisions with family members and loved ones and explain the reasons behind their choices. Although having this conversation may not be easy, it's important for everyone to know what kind of care the patient wants. If it's too hard to have this talk, it may be helpful to plan a family meeting and invite a social worker or member of the faith community to help guide the discussion.

What are the next steps after advance directives have been completed? Where should advance directives be stored?

A member of a patient's health care team or another professional should review the documents to make sure they're filled out correctly. Most states require that signing of the documents be witnessed. Patients should make copies of the documents and put the originals in a safe but easily accessible place. They should give copies to their doctor, hospital, and family members. People may also want to keep in their wallet a card with a written statement declaring that they have a living will and medical power of attorney and describing where the documents can be found. Some organizations will store advance directives and make them available on the patient's behalf.

Can people change their advance directives?

Yes. The process of discussing and writing advance directives should be ongoing, rather than taking place just once. This way a person can review the documents from time to time and modify them if his or her situation or wishes change. Even after advance directives have been signed, patients can change their minds at any time. To update their documents, patients should talk to their health care providers and loved ones about the new decisions they would like to make. When new advance directives have been signed, the old ones should be destroyed.

Do the legal requirements for advance directives vary from state to state?

Yes. Each state has its own laws regarding advance directives. Therefore, special care should be taken to follow the laws of the state where the patient lives or is being treated. It's possible that a living will or medical power of attorney signed in one state may not be recognized in another.

What can caregivers do if advance directives cannot be found and patients can't communicate their wishes?

If decisions about care haven't been discussed between the patient and caregivers in advance, caregivers may feel anxious as they struggle to make these choices for their loved one. It's common for conflicts to develop between family members who have differing opinions. Caregivers may find the following tips helpful:

- Hold a family meeting to talk about the options. Ask the health care team to suggest an expert to guide the discussion.
- Ask the health care team to explain the goals of the medical procedures that are being offered. For example, are the procedures meant to stop the cancer? Lessen pain? Keep the patient alive, and if so, for how long? Caregivers need to know why certain options for care are being offered.
- Think about what the patient would want. Caregivers can imagine what their loved one would say if they could speak at that moment. Did the patient say something in the past that would help with the decision-making process now?

Where can people get help filling out advance directives?

The organizations listed below can help people complete their advance directives. A doctor or nurse, hospital administrator, or social worker may be able to provide assistance as well. Also, although people don't need to hire a lawyer when they want to complete advance directives, a lawyer can explain terms and procedures.

Aging with Dignity

1–888–594–7437 (5WISHES)

850–681–2010

fivewishes@agingwithdignity.org

www.agingwithdignity.org

Aging with Dignity, a national nonprofit organization, worked with the American Bar Association's Commission on Law and Aging to develop an easy-to-read living will called Five Wishes that is legal in 42 states and the District of Columbia. Five Wishes is available in 26 languages, including Spanish and Braille. The organization has also created an advance care planning guide for adolescents and young adults called Voicing My Choices. Both resources can be accessed online or ordered in hard copy format.

Cancer Legal Resource Center

1–866–843–2572 (1–866–THE–CLRC)

CLRC@LLS.edu

www.cancerlegalresourcecenter.org

The Cancer Legal Resource Center (CLRC) is a joint program of the Disability Rights Legal Center and Loyola Law School, Los Angeles. The CLRC provides free information and resources on cancer-related legal issues to people with cancer, survivors, caregivers, employers, health care professionals, and others coping with cancer. The CLRC has a national toll-free line where callers can receive information about relevant laws and resources for their particular situation. A volunteer panel of attorneys and other professionals provides more in-depth information and counsel to CLRC callers. The CLRC provides services in Spanish and has bilingual staff that can assist people on the toll-free line. Some publications are also available in Spanish.

National Hospice and Palliative Care Organization

1–800–658–8898 (helpline)

1–877–658–8896 (multilingual line)

caringinfo@nhpco.org

www.caringinfo.org

The National Hospice and Palliative Care Organization (NHPCO) represents programs and professionals that provide hospice and palliative care in the United States. Caring Connections is a national consumer and community engagement program of NHPCO that works to improve care at the end of life. Caring Connections provides a toll-free number, website, and a wide range of free materials about end-of-life care (such as hospice and palliative care information, advance care planning, and caregiving). Caring Connections provides free advance directives with instructions for each state. Some Spanish-language publications are available, and staff can answer calls in Spanish.

Other MedicalCenter.com Publications

The Key Facts on Arthritis

The Key Facts on Breast Cancer

The Key Facts on Medicare

The Key Facts on Alzheimer's Disease

The Key Facts on Caring For Someone With

Alzheimer's Disease

The Key Facts on Cancer Series

All Titles Can Be Found at

www.Amazon.com

www.MedicalCenter.com

www.ingramcontent.com/pod-product-compliance
Lightning Source LLC
Chambersburg PA
CBHW070549290526
45790CB00002B/616